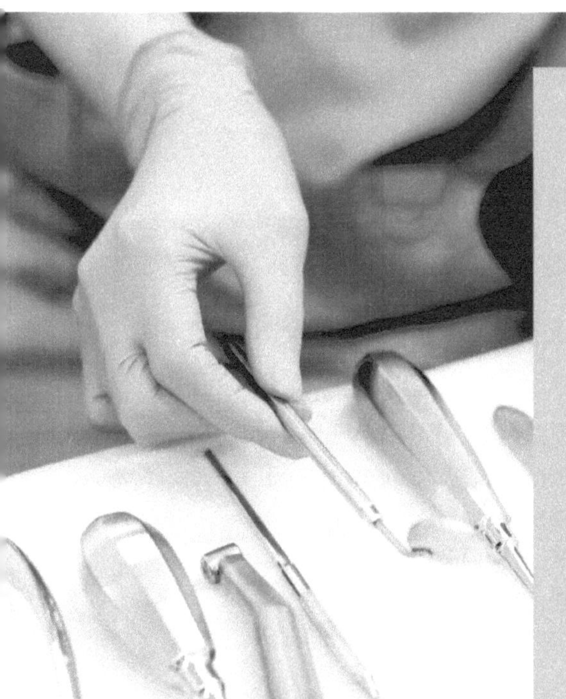

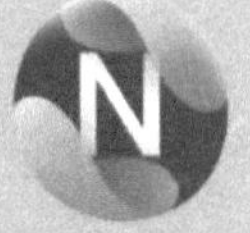

CONTEMPORARY
ANAESTHETIC EQUIPMENT'S

(An aid for healthcare professionals).

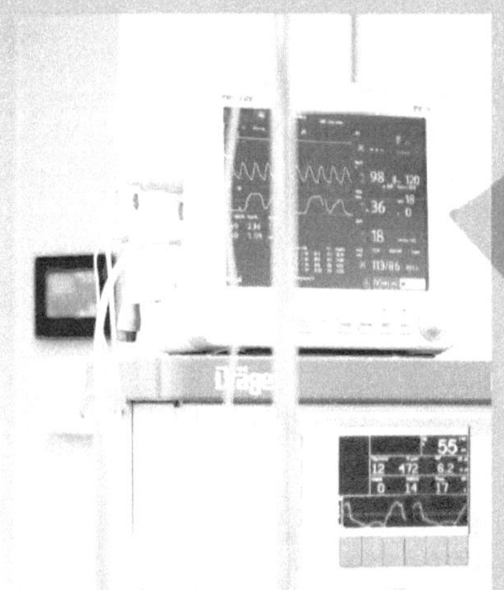

Joshua Jataunamo Oscar

CONTEMPORARY

ANAESTHETIC EQUIPMENTS.

AN AID FOR HEALTHCARE PROFESSIONALS.

First Published, 2023

ISBN: 978-1-304-99639-8

Noogul Digital Publishing

Table of Contents

List of Figures

SECTION ONE:
EQUIPMENT'S USED IN
ANAESTHESIOLOGY

Introduction

The anaesthetic machine enables to deliver gas and vapour mixtures to the patient accurately and continuously. The Boyle anaesthetic machine is designed by **HEG**. Boyle in 1915. Modern machine differs greatly in detail and modified time-to-time, but the basic principles remain the same. It consists of:

    i.   Oxygen and anaesthetic gas supply
    ii.   Pressure gauges
    iii.   Reducing valves
    iv.   Flow meters
    v.   Vapourizers
    vi.   Common gas outlet
    vii.   Certain other features:

High flow oxygen flush, pressure relief valve, oxygen supply failure alarm, suction apparatus! Monitoring devices.

Medical Gas Supply

Cylinders

- Made of molybdenum steel to withstand high pressures
- Made of different sizes (A to J). Size E cylinders are used in the anaesthetic machine
- Oxygen is stored as gas at about 2000 lb/inch^2 and nitrous oxide is stored in a liquid phase with vapour on the top at a pressure of 760 lb/inch^2. It is 75% filled with liquid nitrous oxide **Note:**

Filling ratio is the weight of fluid in the cylinder divided by the weight of water need to fill the cylinder.

- Cylinders are colour coded.
    - Oxygen: Black with white shoulders, green in some countries.
    - Nitrous oxide: Blue
    - Carbon dioxide: Grey
    - Entonox: Blue with white /bluequarters shoulder
    - Air: Grey with white/black quarters shoulder.
- Some markings engraved on the cylinders: Test pressure, chemical formula, Tare weight, dates of test performed, etc.
- Checking and testing by manufacturers at regular intervals:
    - Flattening test
    - Bending test
    - Impact test
    - Pressure test
    - Tensile test.
- Gases and vapour must be free from water vapour as it may freeze and block the exit port at a decreased temperature particularly when opening
- Cylinder valve provides *pin index- system* as a safety feature to make it almost impossible to connect a cylinder to a wrong yoke
- Should be stored in a dry, well-ventilated and fire proof room. Avoid dampness, corrosives and fumes nearby. No oil or grease or any other flammable materials or any source of heat ; should be allowed
- Full cylinders should be kept separately and should not be mixed with empty ones
- Avoid over pressurized full cylinders..

Pin index system

A specific pin configuration for each medical gas on the yoke of the anaesthetic machine. The pin will match the holes on the valve block. It permits only the correct gas cylinder to be fitted in the yoke.

- Oxygen: 2 and 5
- Nitrous oxide: 3 and 5
- Cyclopropane: 3 and 6
- Entonox: 7
- Air: 1 and 5
- Carbon dioxide: 1 and 6

Pressure in the cylinders
- Oxygen: About 2000 lb/inch^2
- Nitrous oxide: About 750 lb/inch^2
- Cyclopropane: 75 lb/inch^2 [stored in light alloy cylinders as a liquid]
- Carbon dioxide: 720 lb/inch^2.

Cylinder valve

- Mounted on the neck of the cylinder, screwed with threaded connection
- The valve can be opened or closed by an off/on spindle for gas pathway
- Non inter changeable safety device (pin index system) prevents wrong cylinder assembly
- Bodok seal is placed between the valve outlet and yoke of the machine to make the gas tight joint.

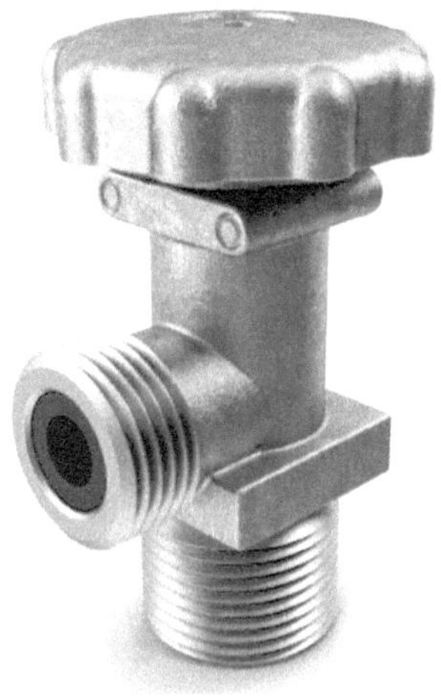

Figure 1: Cylinder Valve Flush Type

- The cylinder valve should be fully open during use. Check the Bodok seal before use to detect any damage.

Piped gas supply

- Gas delivered from a central supply to different locations at a pressure of about 400 kPa;
- Oxygen, nitrous oxide, entonox, compressed air and medical vacuum can be used through the pipe line system
- *Components:*
    - Central supply (cylinder bank/liquid oxygen storage bank or oxygen concentrator)
    - Pipe work (made of copper), flexible and colour coded
    - Outlets (identified by gas colour coding, gas name and by shape) accept matching quid connect or disconnect probes with an indexing colour specific for each gas.

- The cylinders of each group are connected through non return valve to a common pipe. Then in turn *is* connected to the pipe line through pressure regulators
- The cylinders should be well-housed in a well-ventilated room (fire proof) in a suitable place in hospital.

Liquid oxygen

- Oxygen can be stored and supplied in a vacuum thermally insulated evaporator at a temperature of - 150°C to - 170°C and at a pressure of 5 to 10 atmospheres.
- A pressure regulator permits gas to enter the pipelines and maintains it at about 400 kpa
- It also provides a safety valve to release the buildup high pressure, if occurs
- A control valve is also there to meet the extra demands on the system
- Cold oxygen gas is warmed outside the vessel in copper tubing coil. The increase in temperature increases the pressure.

Oxygen Concentrator

- Extracts oxygen from air when exposed a zeolite molecular sieve column at certain pressure.
- The zeolite sieve selectively retains nitrogen and other unwanted constituents of air and releases them to atmosphere
- Maximum oxygen concentration can be-achieved is nearly 95% by volume. Argon may be main of the other constituents.

Compressed Air

- Can be used either clinically at a pressure of 400 kPa or to drive power tools at a pressure of about 700 kPa
- Can be supplied from cylinders or from a compressor
- For clinical use air should be cleaned by filters and separators and then dried.

Pressure Gauge

- Measures the pressure in the cylinder mounted in the front facing panel on the anaesthetic machine
- High pressure gas acts to straighten a coiled tube (Bourdon gauge). Movement of the tube causes the needle pointer to move on a calibrated dial to indicate the pressure

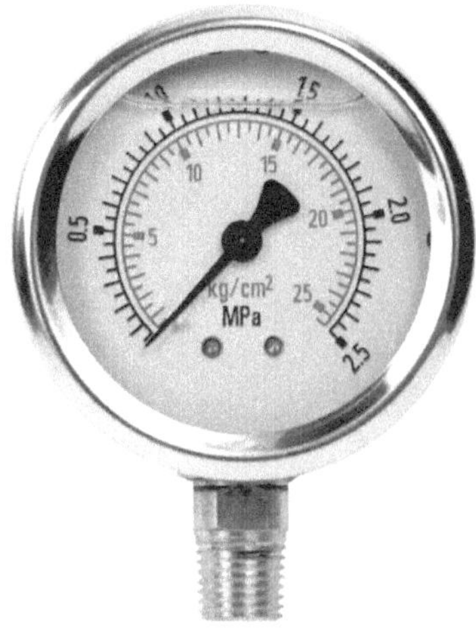

Figure 2: Pressure Gauge

- Colour coded and calibrated for a particular gas or vapour
- Indicates the contents of gas available in the cylinder
- Nitrous oxide cylinder does not provide pressure gauge as it is stored as a *liquid* and vapour
- Pressure gauge meant for pipeline is not for cylinder and *vice versa.* May lead to inaccuracies and/or damage
- Misassemble is possible.

Pressure regulator (Reducing valve)
- Reduces the variable gas pressure from cylinders to about 400 kpa
- Positioned between the cylinders and the rest of anaesthesia machine
- Provides fine control of gas flow and protects the parts of machine against high pressure
- Prevents the pressure from increasing above a predetermined limit
- Contents of the cylinder should be free from water, otherwise ice can form inside the valve
- Earlier models are with 'fins' to augment acquisition of heat from the environment
- Mechanism of action: The gas from the cylinder enters into the chamber of reducing valve where it distorts a diaphragm to which a toggle mechanism is connected and a balance between two opposing forces maintains a constant predetermined operating pressure (60 psi)
- Diaphragm can rupture
- Relief valve is fitted downstream of the regulator. It helps to escape the gas, if regulator fails.

Flow restrictor
- Pipeline pressure increase can be controlled by using a pressure regulator on a flow restrictor
- Flow restrictor provides a constriction between the pipeline supply and the remaining part of the anaesthetic machine. The constriction causes a significant pressure drop in presence of a high gas flow rate.

Flowmeters
- Measures flow rate of a gas per minute
- Each gas is individually calibrated

- Oxygen should be the last to be added in mixture
- Calibration done at room temperature and atmospheric pressure, accuracy with an error margin ±2%
- It contains: A flow control valve, a tapered (wider at the top) transparent glass or plastic tube, a light weight rotating bobbin. Bobbin stops at either end of the tube
- Flow control (needle) valves:
  - Controls the flow through the flow meters by manual adjustment
  - Positioned at the base of flow meter
  - Control knobs are labelled and colour coded, blue for nitrous oxides, white for oxygen and grey for carbon dioxide.

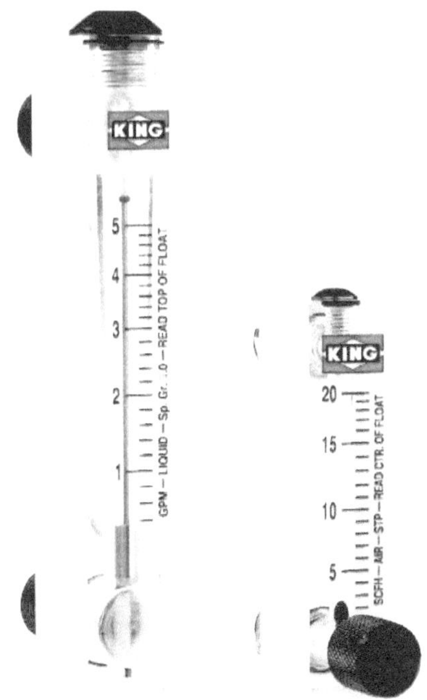

- When the gas flows, with the help of flutes the bobbin spins clears of the walls of the tube and thus avoids the errors of friction. Bobbins should be made antistatic
- The viscosity and density of the gases can influence the gas flow in the flow meter. Each flow meter is calibrated for each gas
- Flow meter should be set in vertical position, otherwise may give incorrect reading
- Malfunction: Broken, cracked, bobbin stuck, wrong gas, improper alignment, back pressure, etc.
- Other types:
  - Heidbrink flow meter: Metal tapered tube with inverted black float
  - Connell flow meter: Provides round float, reading from its center.

Vapourizers

To administer a controlled amount of an inhalational agent after changing a liquid to vapour to fresh gas flow.

Ideal vapourizers characteristics
- Performance not affected by changes in fresh gas flow, liquid volume, ambient temperature, land pressure, decrease in temperature due to vaporization and pressure fluctuation due to |mode of respiration
- *Low* resistance to flow
- Light weight with small liquid requirement
- Economy, safety, minimum servicing
- Corrosion and solvent resistant
- Quality control by authorized institution.

Boyle anaesthetic machine provides two vaporizing bottles one for diethyl ether and the other \ for trichlorethylene. These vapourizers are of variable bypass, flow over or bubble through type. These are neither properly calibrated nor temperature compensated. (Bodman R, Gillies D. Harold Griffith. , 1992)

The concentration of vapour depends on the rate of gas flow, liquid surface area, the way the gas impinges on the liquid and the temperature of liquid.

Boyle's bottle/glass-ether vapourizers
- Contains diethyl ether which vaporizes to an extent governed by its saturated vapour pressure; at room temperature
- The amount of gas entering the vapourizer can be altered by moving the lever
- Gas enters the vapourizer above the anaesthetic liquid to vaporize and its concentration c be altered by depressing the plunger
- Vapourization needs latent heat of Vapourization. Larger amount of heat is needed to vaporize ether. The concentration from the vapourizer usually falls significantly as the temperature are vapour pressure of ether fall. So the total gas flow may need to pass through the vapourize) and even bubbled through it.
- Sealing washer of the Boyle's bottle should be of good order
-

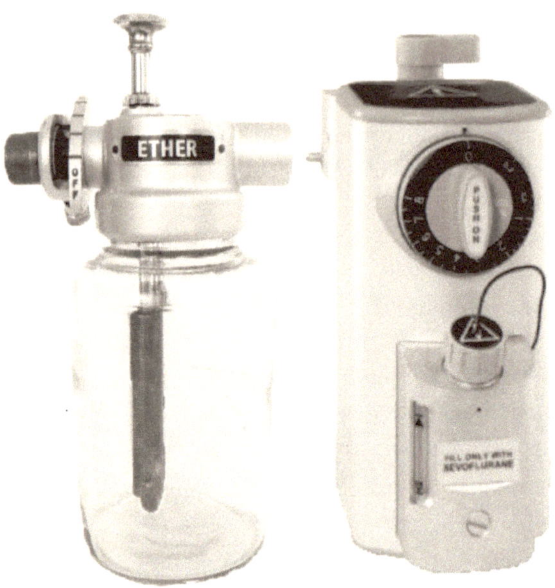

Figure 4: Boyles Ether / Isofluorane Vaporiser

- Dark brown-coloured bottles are used as ether can be decomposed by light
- Metal parts of U tube and hood of plunger should be made of copper as it is anticatalyst and can prevent decomposition of ether.

Trichloroethylene vapourizer bottle

It is similar to ether bottle but it is smaller in size and the inlet U tube and the hood of plunger *are* entirely chrome plated.

Goldman halothane vapourizer

- Simple vapourizer, flow-over type, no wicks
- Neither temperature compensated, not accurately calibrated
- Can be used inside or outside the breathing circuit

- Control device on the top which can be rotated to alter the vapourizer output
- Low resistance to gas flow
- Maximum concentration never exceeds 3%
- Vapour concentration can be increased by
    - Splashing
    - Incorporating wicks
    - Employing 2 vapourizers in series.

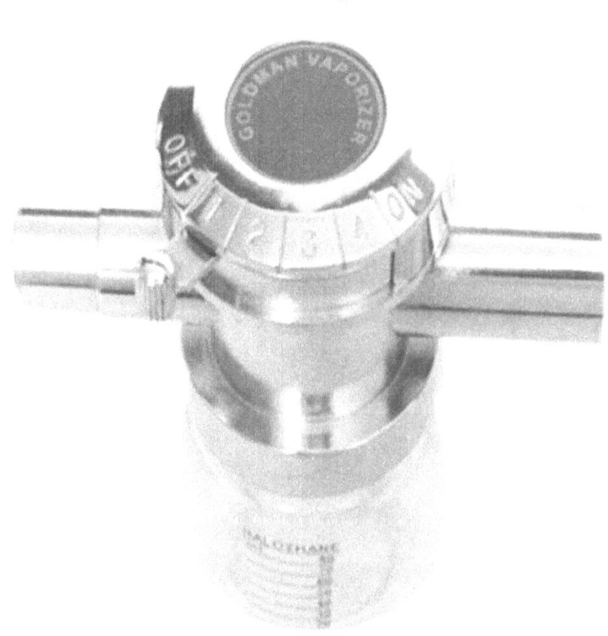

Figure 5: Goldman Vaporizer

Back bar

- Part of the Boyle machine on which rota meter (containing flow meters), vapourizers (ether and trichloroethylene) and other accessories are fitted
- *Trilene safety interlock'* is placed at the end of back bar
- Provides an angled outlet with a non return valve to prevent a back pressure during positive pressure ventilation
- At extreme right there is an *emergency by pass* which can deliver high flow of Oxygen (O_2) directly, by passing the rota meter

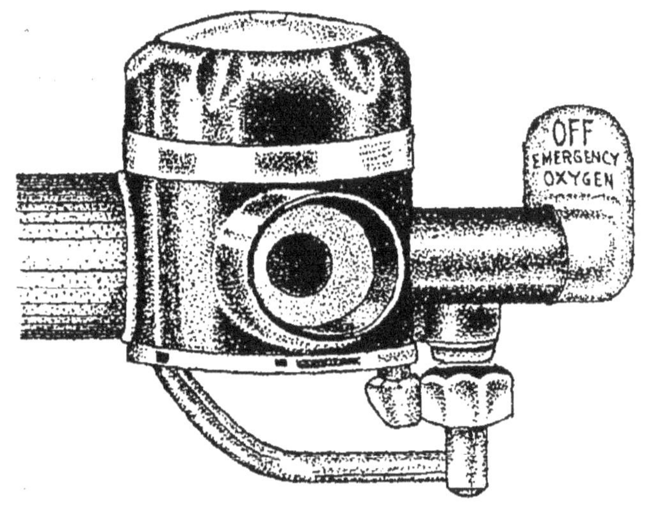

Figure 6: Trilene Interlock Unit

- Some machines may have an emergency press button unit to supply plentiful oxygen (oxygen flush). Risk of accidental activation includes barotrauma, dilution of anaesthetic gas awareness.

Oxygen supply failure alarm

- Various designs are available
- Activates on the pressure of oxygen
- No need of battery or mains power
- Gives audible signal sufficient to draw attention
- Should have pressure linked control which interrupt the flow of other gases when they come into operation.

Plenum vapourizers

- Designed to maintain a constant output of volatile anaesthetic agent
- The case is made of copper which is a good heat sink
- Provides a bypass channel and vapourizing chamber which contains wicks to increase surface area available for Vapourization
- Has a temperature-compensation device. Bimetallic strip inside to compensate for the cooling of the liquid anaesthetic. When cooling takes place due to latent heat of vaporization, the string made of two different metals with different coefficients of expansion bend to permit a greater fraction of the total flow to enter the vapourizing chamber (Brockwell RC, Andrews GG. , 2002)
- The gas coming out of the vapourizing chamber is fully saturated
- The effect of back pressure is compensated
- The calibration of each vapourizer is agent specific
- Vapourizer filling devices are agent specific. These are geometrically coded to fit the safety filling port of the correct vapourizer and anaesthetic bottle. The fillers are also colour coded, *red* halothane, *orange* for enflurane and *purple* for isoflurane.
- *Caution:*

- The liquid anaesthetic should not enter the bypass channel
- The effect of back pressure must be compensated
- Preservative like thymol (in halothane) can deposit on wicks and interfere the efficacy of vapourizer. Enflurane and isoflurane do not contain preservative
- A pressure relief valve can prevent the damage of flow meter/vapourizer
- Corrosion of bimetallic strip can occur.

Common gas outlet
- Receives all gases and vapours from the machine
- Attached to the delivery hose
- Leak /disconnection can occur. Adequate care is needed
- A check valve can be provided just proximal to outlet to prevent retrograde gas flow from flush valve or breathing system.

Bag mount
- Made of metal or Plastic tube. One end connected with machine outflow and the other end to the angle piece adaptor to connect corrugated rubber hose. Rebreathing bag is attached from the under surface
- May have a valve. By turning a lever to one side, the rebreathing bag is cut out of the circuit
- In intermittent flow machine the bag and bag mount should be removed from the machine.

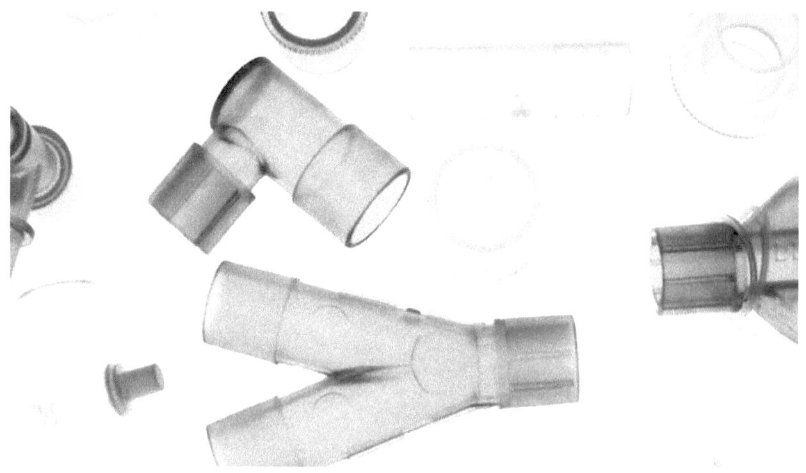

Figure 7: A Bag Mount

Rebreathing bag

- Made of antistatic rubber, ellipsoidal in shape
- Capacity may vary from $2L$ to 0.5L, capacity of bag must exceed patient's tidal volume. Accommodates fresh gas flow
- Bag movement is important in assessing or controlling the ventilation
- Limits pressure build up in the system
- Must be comfortable for use.

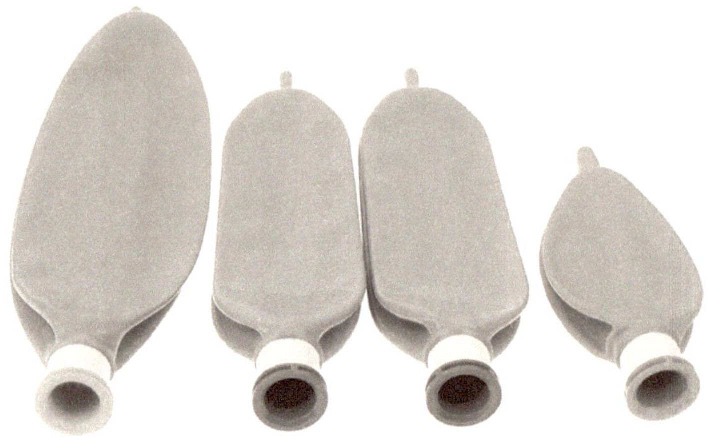

Figure 8: Rebreathing / Reservoir Bag

Corrugated Rubber Tube
- Flexible, light weight breathing tube. Made of antistatic rubber. Usual length about 1 meter
- Corrugation helps acute angulation without kinking
- Can act as reservoir in certain systems
- Can be used to connect the ventilator to the breathing circuit
- Tube diameter should be such to present low resistance to gas flow and to promote a laminar flow
- Irregular walls of the tube may cause some turbulence and allow some dirt or infective material into it.

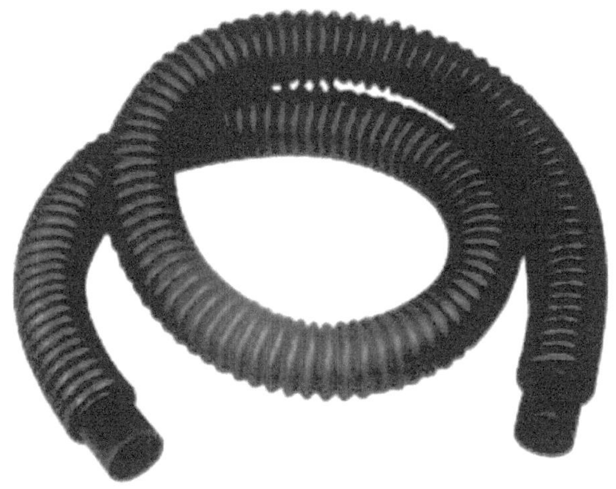

Adjustable pressure limiting valve (Expiratory valve)

- Allows the exhaled gas and excess fresh gas flow out of the breathing system
- One way spring loaded valves with three ports: Inlet, patient and exhaust ports. The exhaust port can be open to atmosphere
- The spring adjusts the pressure required to open the valve
- During spontaneous ventilation, a positive pressure in the system during expiration can cause the valve to open
- During positive pressure ventilation an intentional leak is produced by adjusting the valve dial during inspiration

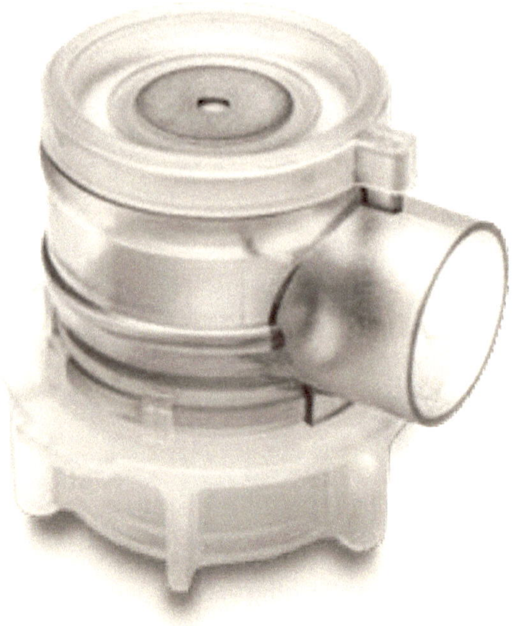

Figure 10: Expiratory Valve

- Malfunction:
    - May remain opened/closed.
    - If closed, a pressure relief safety mechanism should be there which is activated at a pressure of about 60 cm H_2O
    - Condensation of water vapour can damage the valve.

Face mask and angle piece
- Made of antistatic rubber or transparent plastic designed to fit the contour of face anatomically
- Air filled cuff ensures the snug fit over the face
- Proximal end connects to the angle piece
- May have some clamps for the harness to be attached

- It should have a minimum dead space. Dead space may increase by up to 200 ml in adults
- Problems:
    - Difficult to achieve airtight seal over the face particularly in edentulous patients
    - Excessive pressure by mask can damage branches of trigeminal or facial nerve.

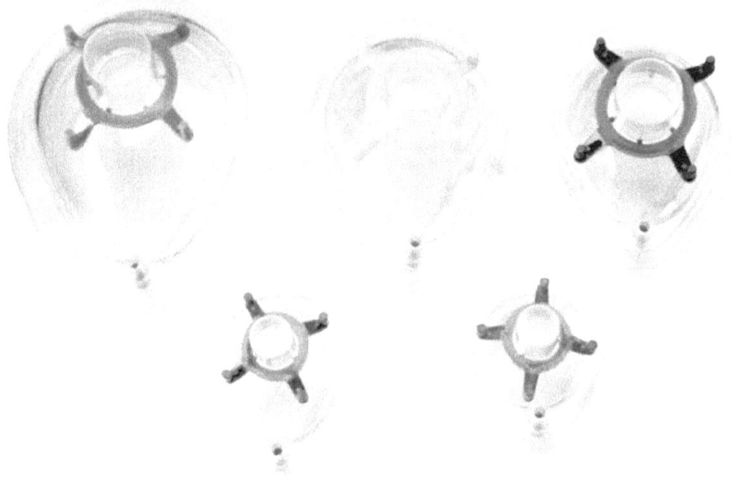

Figure 11: Anaesthesia Face Masks

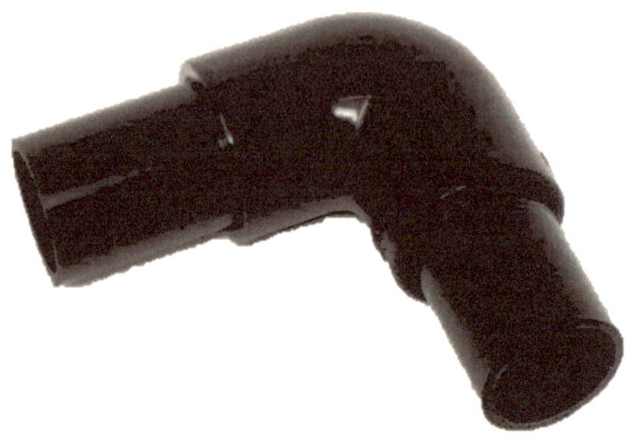

Figure 12: Face Mask Angle Piece Adaptor

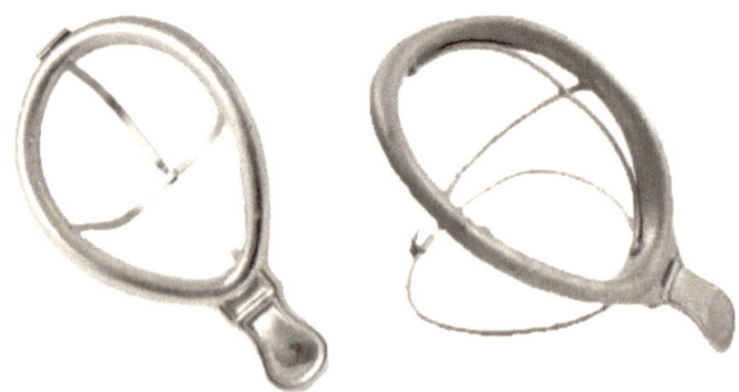

Figure 13: Schimmelbusch Mask

Anaesthetic Breathing System
Formerly classified as open, semi open, semi closed and closed systems.

- Open system (open drop inhalation method):

- Volatile anaesthetic is administered to the patient with atmospheric air. Respiratory tract has access to atmosphere all the time during both inspiration and expiration
- No reservoir/rebreathing bag
- Schimmelbusch mask is used for open drop anaesthesia. It consists of a simple wire frame over which 8 to 12 layers of gauge are stretched and kept in position. Mask provides one effective surface for volatile anaesthetics and some space for confining the anaesthetic vapour.
- Semi open system: Here also the anaesthetic is administered with air and respiratory tract is open to atmosphere during inspiration and expiration. But some reservoir is made over the mask (by a folded towel over the mask), but it is mostly open to the atmosphere
- Semi closed system:
  - Patient inhales from the continuous flow of gases/vapours from anaesthetic machine and, it includes one reservoir/rebreathing bag
  - When all the expired gases escape to the atmosphere through non rebreathing valve, then , it is non-rebreathing type of semi closed system
  - If part of exhaled gases escape through expiratory valve and part passes through rebreathing bag then it is partial rebreathing type of semi closed system.
- Closed system:
  - Anaesthetic gases and vapours are not voided in atmosphere. The same gases are continuously recycled after absorption of carbon dioxide by soda lime.
  - Oxygen utilized in metabolism and gases/vapours utilized in the body or lost are to be supplemented
  - Some intentional leak is always kept in expiratory valve.

Advantages:

i. Economy
ii. Retention of body heat and moisture
iii. Less pollution
iv. Less chance of explosion.

Disadvantages:

i. Circuit should be leak proof
ii. Cumbersome and heavy equipment
iii. CO_2 absorption may not be adequate
iv. Resistance to breathing and dead space may be high
v. Heat from soda lime may affect the body
vi. Alkaline dust from soda lime may also affect the body
vii. Cross infection
viii. Dilution of fresh gas mixture possible.

Soda Lime

Composition: Sodium hydroxide 4%

Potassium hydroxide 1% Water 14 to 19%

Silica (to prevent powdering calcium hydroxide) 95%

4 to 8 mesh

Conical neutralization of CO_2

$$CO_2 + H_2O \rightarrow H_2CO_3$$
$$H_2CO_3 + 2NaOH \rightarrow Na_2CO_3 + 2H_2O + heat$$
$$H_2CO_3 + Ca(OH)_2 \rightarrow CaCO_3 + 2H_2O + heat$$

- Soda lime is pink coloured and it turns white when it becomes ineffective. There is gain in weight, when it is exhausted. Some regeneration can occur, when it is rested for 2 to 3 hours

- Trichloroethylene should never be used in a closed circuit with soda lime, otherwise toxic products dichloroacetylene may be formed. It can produce paralysis of cranial nerves particularly 5th and 7th cranial nerve.

Baralyme

Composition: Barium hydroxide 20%
                 Calcium hydroxide 80%
                 Water bound crystallization
                 No silica is needed,
Chemical neutralization of CO_2

$$CO_2 + H_2O \rightarrow H_2CO_3$$
$$H_2CO_3 + Ba(OH)_2 \rightarrow BaCO_3 + 2H_2O + heat$$
$$H_2CO_3 + Ca(OH)_2 \rightarrow CaCO_3 + 2H_2O$$

- Produces less heat than soda lime
- Less caustic than soda lime.

Absorbers

- Absorber of to-and-fro system is made of metal, but that of circle system is usually glass or transparent plastic. Metals conduct and dissipate heat better and more resistant to corrosive effects of alkali. Plastic *is* light and enables to observe -colour changes
- Shape cylindrical. Wide and short canister preferred
- Granular space: Space occupied by the absorbent. Measure by the bulk density. *It* is 0.9 gm/ cc for soda lime and 1 gm/cc for baralyme
- Air space: Usually 45 to 75% of the volume of canister. It includes inter granular (void) space and intra granular (pore) space
- Inter granular space: Usually about *45%*, depends of size of granules and type of packaging
- Intra granular space: Space within the pores of granules. Vary directly with the weight of absorbent but inversely with its moisture content. Usually about *25ml/100gm* of absorbent.

- Exhaustion time depends on exhaled CO_2, type of ventilation, tidal volume, and absorbent capacity, degree of channeling, fresh gas flow, position and accuracy of the canister.

Water's 'to-and-fro' system

- Introduced by Ralph Waters in *1923*
- A soda lime canister is place between the face mask and rebreathing bag. Both inspiration and expiration take place through the canister. Fresh gas should be very near to face mask.

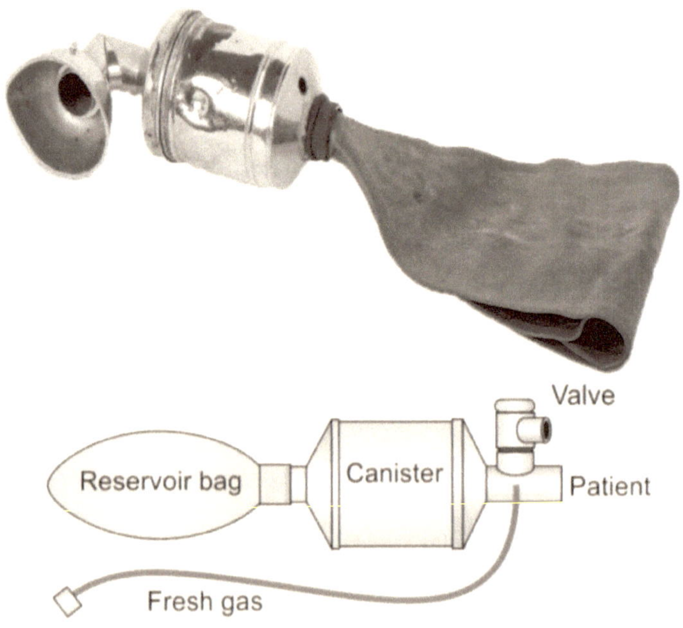

Figure 14: Dr. Ralph Waters To and Fro System Canister

- Canister: 8x13 cm, capacity 1 Ib soda *lime*. Air space about 400 ml, inter granular space should be nearly the tidal volume of the patient
- Resistance of this circuit may be more than 2 to 3 cm H_2O during spontaneous ventilation
- Mechanical dead space: About 200 ml (from wire gauge of canister to face)
- Channeling can occur. Canister needs adequate proper filling
- Disadvantages: Heat production, alkaline dust, channeling, reduced efficiency
- Advantages: Cheap, simple, easy to operate and sterilize, low resistance, conservation of moisture and heat.

Circle breathing system
- Soda lime is used to absorb the patient's exhaled CO2- Fresh gas flow requirement is low
- Soda lime canister is positioned vertically. It provides an inlet delivering fresh gas flow from machine and 2 ports — one to deliver fresh gas flow to patients and the other to receive exhaled gases from the patient. These 2 ports incorporate unidirectional valve. An expiratory valve connected to a rebreathing bag.
- Inspiratory and expiratory tubing's are connected to the canister
- A vapourizer can be incorporated in the back bar of the anaesthetic machine (outside circle) or on the expiratory limb within the circle (VIC)

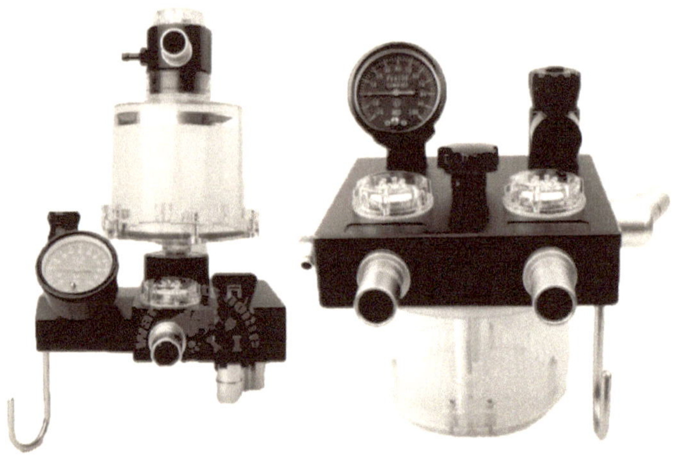

Figure 15: Circle Carbon dioxide Absorber

- Exhaled gases are circled back to the soda lime canister. After CO_2 absorption the gas joins the fresh gas flow to be delivered to patient
- The system can be used for both spontaneous or controlled ventilation
- Mechanical dead space includes the space between the face piece and the beginning of double corrugated tubing. Resistance to gases is within 2 to 3 cm H_2O pressure
- Canister usually large, capacity 41b soda lime, divided in two halves and this is reversible
- Advantages: Efficient
- Disadvantages: Bulkiness, more resistance, more difficulty in recharging, chance of cross infection
- Malfunction: Expiratory valve stuck closed, inspiratory valve stuck closed, circle system valve stuck open, misassembled valve components, foreign body in valve assembly

- Adequate monitoring of inspired oxygen, end tidal CO_2 and inhalation anaesthetic needed.

Vapourizer outside the circle breathing system
- Positioned on the back bar
- Can deliver high output concentration at low flow rates
- Have high resistance to gas flow
- Vapourizers should be efficient enough to deliver proper concentration of vapour with both high and low fresh gas flows.

Vapourizer inside the circle breathing system
- Minimal resistance to gas flow
- Positioned in the expiratory limb
- Here vapour-free fresh gas flow dilutes the inspired vapour concentration
- During spontaneous ventilation, deep anaesthesia depresses respiration and thus anaesthetic uptake is reduced and overdose of anaesthetic is prevented. This mechanism is absent in controlled ventilation.

Mapleson Classification

Mapleson classified the breathing system as Mapleson A, B, C, D, E and F. Nodaway's only A D, E and F and some of their modifications are in common use.

Criteria for an Ideal Breathing System

- Simple and easy to use
- Safe and efficient
- Can be used in all age groups
- Can be used in either spontaneous or controlled ventilation
- Satisfactory with low fresh gas flow

- No complications like barotrauma
- Compact, lightweight, cheap, minimum running cost, easy to maintain
- Can be easily sterilized
- Easy removal of exhaled gas possible.

Mapleson A System

- Mostly popular and widely used
- Contains a fresh gas inlet connected to a reservoir bag, then attached to a corrugated tube and then connected with face mask or endotracheal tube

Figure 16: Mapleson A Circuit

- Not ideal for controlled/assisted ventilation. Can be used for spontaneous ventilation. Fresh: gas flow should be equal to alveolar minute volume (about 10 ml/kg/min)
- Rebreathing occurs and not suitable for Intermittent Positive Pressure Ventilation (IPPV) unless large fresh gas flow is used
- Most commonly used version of Mapleson A is Magill system
- Not ideal for Paediatric anaesthesia. (Aridi M, Hussein B, Hajj-Hassan M, Khachfe HM. , 2016)

Mapleson B System

- Fresh gas inlet is towards patient end in between the expiratory valve and corrugated tube. Contains a reservoir bag at one end of tubing and face mask/endotracheal tube as usual
- Less efficient during spontaneous ventilation, but more efficient in controlled ventilation
- Not used commonly

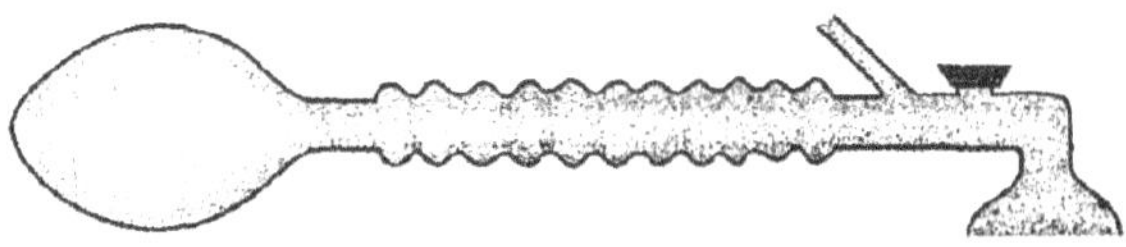

Figure 17: Mapleson B Circuit

Mapleson C System

- Mostly similar to Mapleson B system
- Here corrugated tube is absent. Reservoir bag is attached to fresh gas inlet. Expiratory valve is in between face mask/endotracheal tube and fresh gas inlet
- Not much used.

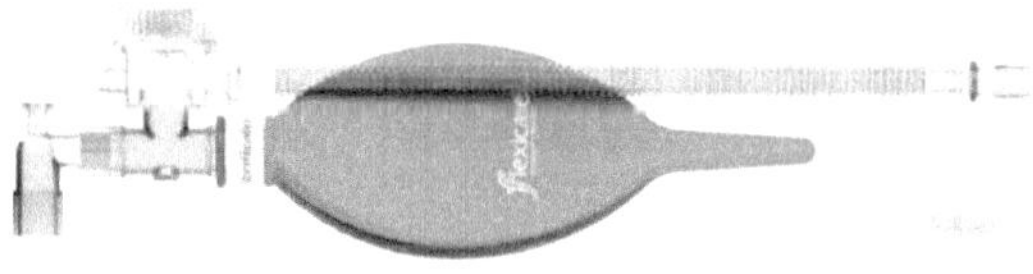

Figure 18: Mapleson C Circuit

Mapleson D System

- Consists of face mask/endotracheal tube, fresh gas inlet nearer face mask, corrugated tube and connected with expiratory valve and reservoir bag
- Efficient for controlled/assisted ventilation. Can be used in spontaneous ventilation
- Bain coaxial system is the modification of Mapleson D system.

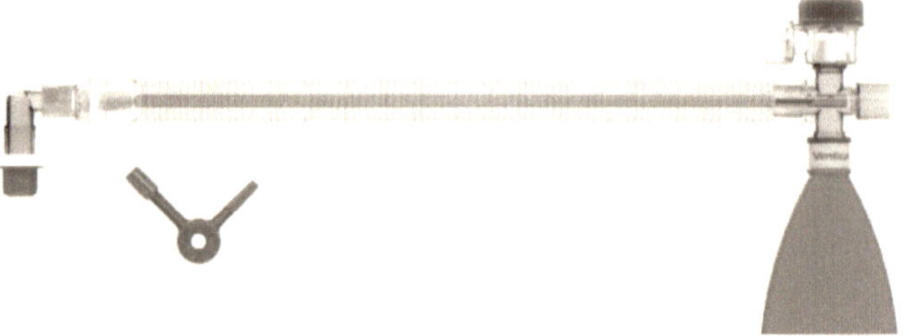

Figure 19: Mapleson D Circuit

Mapleson E System

- Identical with Ayre's T piece system
- Fresh gas flow is nearer to face mask/endotracheal tube, then connected to corrugated tube
- No reservoir bag is used. No expiratory valve is there
- It is a T-piece with 3 ports, Fresh gas flow in one port, second port to face mask, third port is meant for tubing
- Widely used in Paediatric anaesthesia (up to 25 kg body weight)
- Needs high fresh gas flow to prevent rebreathing
- As there is no expiratory valve in this system, scavenging is a problem.

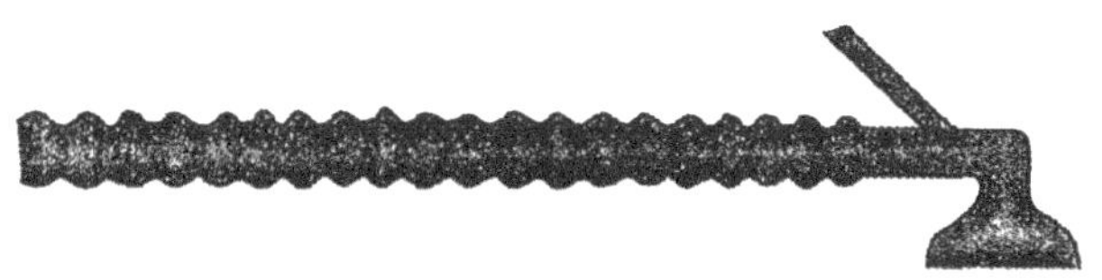

Figure 20: Mapleson E Circuit

Mapleson F System

- Modified version of Mapleson E system
- Here in T-piece system a double ended bag is attached to the end of the tubing
- Suitable for spontaneous/controlled ventilation Widely used in Paediatric anaesthesia (up to 25 kg)
- Needs high fresh gas flow (2.5 to 3 times minute ventilation) to prevent rebreathing
- Volume of reservoir bag should approximate tidal volume.

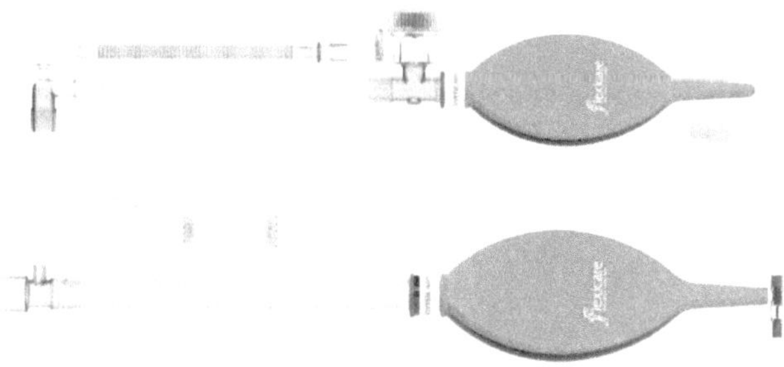

Figure 21: Mapleson F Circuit

Bain Circuit

- Coaxial version of Mapleson D system
- Fresh gas flow through inner tube, exhaled gas through outer tube. The reservoir bag and *expiratory* valve mounted at the machine end
- Internal tube should have swivel mount at patient end to avoid kinking
- Tubes are transparent to detect inside, and kinking, or disconnection
- Efficient in controlled ventilation. Fresh gas flow rate should be 70 to 100 ml/kg/min
- Not much efficient for spontaneous ventilation. Fresh gas flow should be 200 to 300 ml/kg to prevent rebreathing

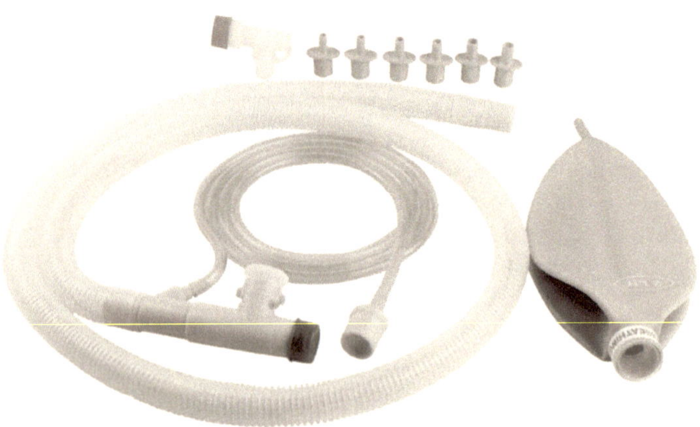

Figure 22: Bain Circuit

- Use of ventilator is possible in this system
- Usual length 180 cm

- Advantages: Simple, light weight and easy to handle, safe and reliable. Can be easily sterilized, disposable tubing available
- Disadvantages: Unrecognized disconnection, kinking, etc.

Endotracheal Tubes and Airways

Endotracheal tubes

- Tubes through which the anaesthetic gas/vapours along with respiratory gases are conveyed to and from the trachea. It is the artificial extension of larynx and a means of securing the airway
- Two ends: Patient end is beveled, machine end is not
- Made of plastic (disposable) or red rubber or latex
- Criteria for an ideal endotracheal tube: Nontoxic, no allergic, smooth, properly curved, low kink ability, easily sterilized, smooth, cheap
- Oro tracheal tube: Short, curved and bevel angle should not be less than 45° in relation to long axis

- Naso tracheal tube: Long curve, bevel angle should not be less than 30° to long axis
- Size of the tube: Magill system arbitrary number from 00 to widest 10. French scale denotes the external diameter in mm multiplied by 3. It is more or less the external circumference of the tube. Internal diameter of the tube ranges from 4 to 12 mm. Usually 8.5 mm tube is meant for females and 9.5 mm for males.

Length of the tube:

- About twice the length from the ear to his nostrils
- Usually about 24 to 30 cm in adults
- Formula for children: Age (years)/2 + 12 cm for oral tube.

    Age (years)/2 + 15 cm for nasal tube.

- Diameter of the tube in children; 4.5 mm + Age (years)/4 in mm
- Cuff of the endotracheal tube: To provide an airtight endotracheal seal. Consists of an inflating tube and a pilot balloon. Cuff is vulcanized on the outer side of the tube about 12 mm from its end. Usually inflated with 4 to 8 ml air.

An ideal cuff should expand symmetrically and the distance between the end of cuff and the nearest part of the cuff should be 1 to 1.25 cm. Overinflated cuff may cause ulceration and necrosis and even tracheal stenosis.

Type of cuff:

- Low volume cuff: Needs inflation to a high pressure to produce seal. High pressure cuff causes little pressure on tracheal wall

- High volume/low pressure cuff: Usually floppy. May fit an irregularly shaped tracheal wall. Insertion is usually difficult and traumatic
- Sometimes double cuffs are used for alternate inflation and deflation at regular intervals to minimize pressure effect
- Cuff volume should be monitored and readjusted, whenever needed
- N2O may diffuse into the cuff filled with air and thus may increase the pressure
- Avoid cuffed tubes in children.

Oxford endotracheal tube

- L-shaped non kinking endotracheal tube mostly used for head and neck surgery
- Made of rubber/plastic, cuffed or uncuffed, wall is thick
- Bevel is oval-shaped, faces posteriorly

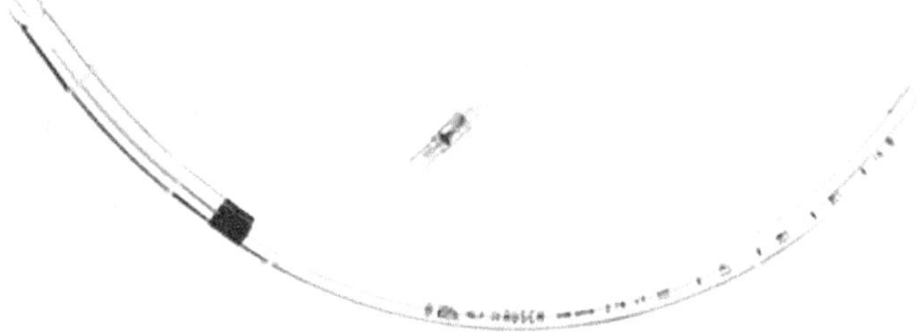

Figure 24: Oxford Non-kinking Endotracheal Tube

- Stylet is needed for its insertion
- Distance from the bevel to the curve of the tube is fixed.

Armoured endotracheal tube

- Made of plastic or silicone
- Thick walls contain a spiral of metal wire or tough nylon
- Spiral helps to prevent kinking
- Introducer is needed for its insertion
- Tube length is fixed; risk of bronchial intubation
- Used in anaesthesia for head/neck surgery.

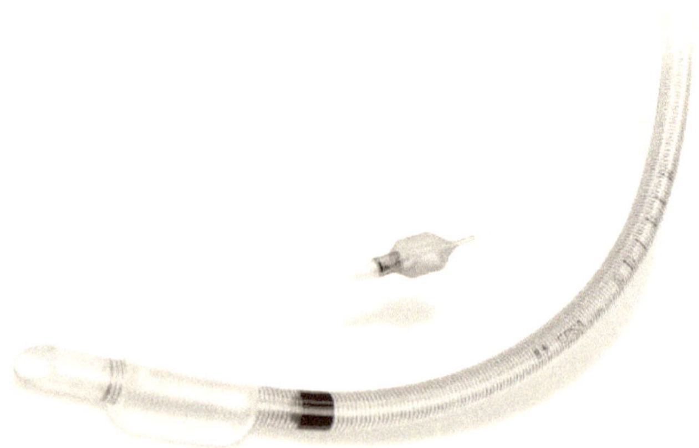

Figure 25: Latex Armoured Endotracheal Tube

RAE (Ring, Adair and Elwyn) endotracheal tube

- Preformed shape to fit the mouth and nose without kinking
- Provides a bend located just as the tube emerges at the level of chin/forehead
- Cuffed/non cuffed variety

- Uncuffed tubes mainly used in Paediatric cases
- Cuffed tube may include one Murphy eye
- Uncuffed tube may contain two Murphy eyes
- Risk of bronchial intubation.

Laser resistant endotracheal tube

- Used for anaesthesia in laser surgery on larynx/trachea
- Designed to withstand the effects of laser beams and thus helps the risk of fire or damages of the tube
- Has a flexible stainless steel body
- Reflected beams from the tube defocussed to reduce the unwanted laser strike to healthy tissues
- Cuff should be filled with saline instead of air to reduce the risks of ignition
- Some designs may have two cuffs. (Kalu Q, Edentekhe TA, Eguma S., 2020)

Micro laryngeal endotracheal tube

- Tube is of small diameter but with an adult sized cuff
- It can be used nasally
- Helps better exposure and surgical access to the larynx.

Tracheostomy tubes

- Curved plastic tubes
- Usually inserted through 2nd, 3rd, and 4th tracheal ring
- Introducer needed for insertion

- Provides wings on the proximal part of the tube to fix
- May be cuffed / uncuffed
- Proximal end ends in a standard 15 mm connector. Tip is cut horizontally
- Different sizes are available
- Uses:
    - Long-term IPPV
    - Upper airway obstruction
    - Maintenance of airway to protect the lungs.

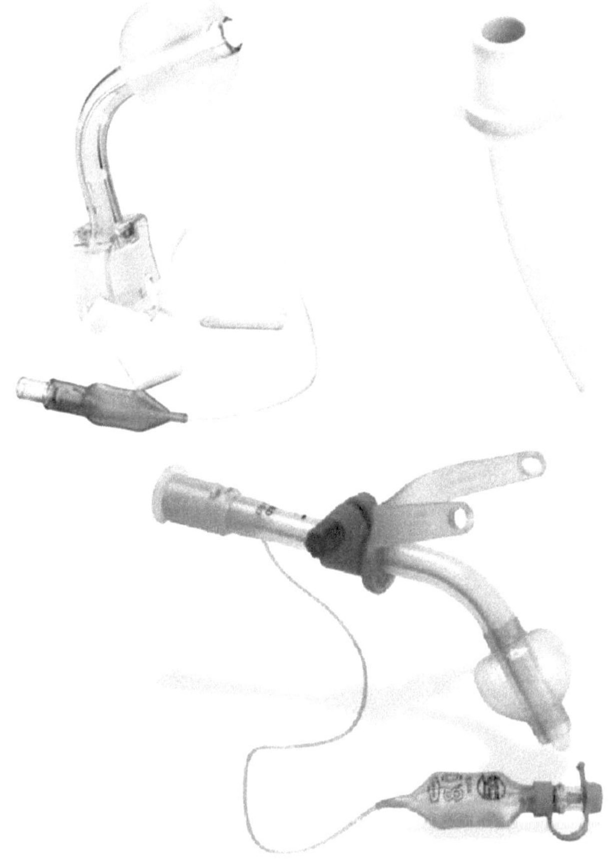

Figure 26: Tracheostomy Tubes Cuffed and Uncuffed

- Side effects:
  - Loss of voice
  - Loss of expulsive cough
  - Loss of nasal humidifying effect.

- Complications:
    - Displacement
    - Accidental bronchial intubation
    - Erosion of vessels
    - Obstruction
    - Tracheal ulceration
    - Tracheal stenosis.

Metal Tracheostomy Tubes

- Made of stainless steel/silver
- Provides inner and outer tube
- Uncuffed

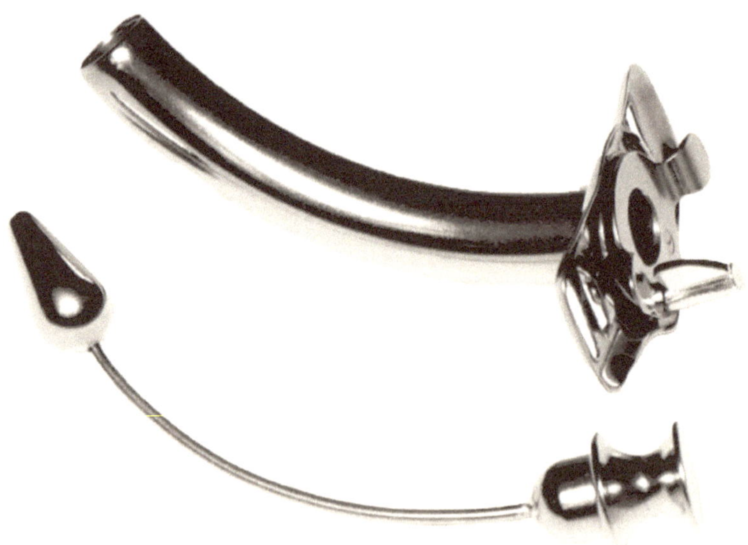

- Inner rube usually removed for clearing at regular intervals
- Used in cases needing long-term IPPV
- After long term use, a track is formed and them the tracheostomy tube is removed
- Speaking version is available.

Double Lumen Endobronchial Tubes

- Allows the anaesthetist to deflate one particular lung while maintaining standard ventilation of the other
- Includes two separate lumens each with its own cuff and pilot tube and balloon
- Contains two curves, anterior and lateral. Anterior curve is usual to fit the upper airway and the lateral curve (right or left) to fit into the right or left bronchus

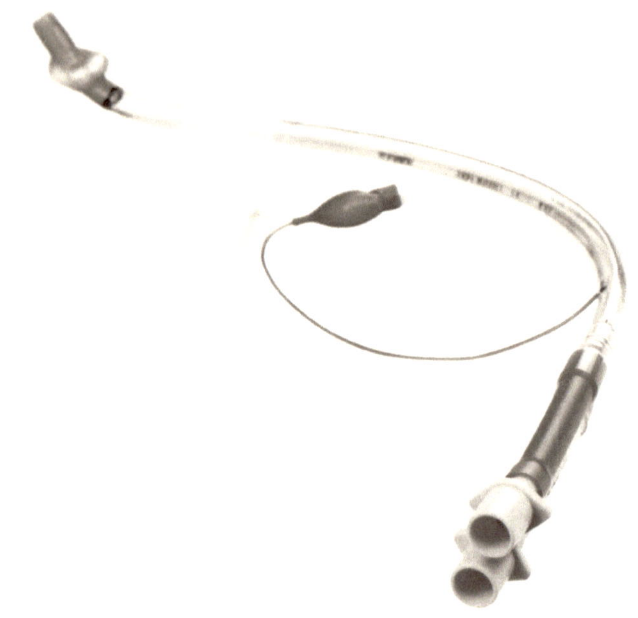

Figure 28: Double Lumen Endobronchial Tube

- The machine end of the tube is connected to a Y-shaped catheter mount to connect the breathing system
- Right sided variety provides an eye in the bronchial cuff to ventilate the right upper lobe. No eyes in left sided variety
- Carlen's tube is commonly used and it has a carina hook. Other varieties: Robertshaw, Dr. White and Sheridan Sheri-I-Bronch endobronchial tubes.
- Tubes are available in various sizes
- Position of the tube must be checked just after intubation and immediately after positioning for surgery
- Problems
    - Hook can cause trauma

- Relatively small lumens cause increase in resistance and difficulty in suctioning
- Needs technical skill and experience
- Risk of malpositioning.

Oropharyngeal Airway

- Curved tubes, anatomically shaped, made of metal or rubber or plastic
- Inserted through the mouth into oropharynx above the tongue to maintain the upper airway patency
- Prevents the fall back of the tongue in an unconscious patient
- Curved body contains air channel. Usually flattened anteroposteriorly and curved laterally
- Flange at the oral end
- Bite part is straight and hard, fits in between the teeth
- Available in various sizes and in different varieties.
  - Philips airway: Rounded rubber tube with a metal mount, flattened on cross section

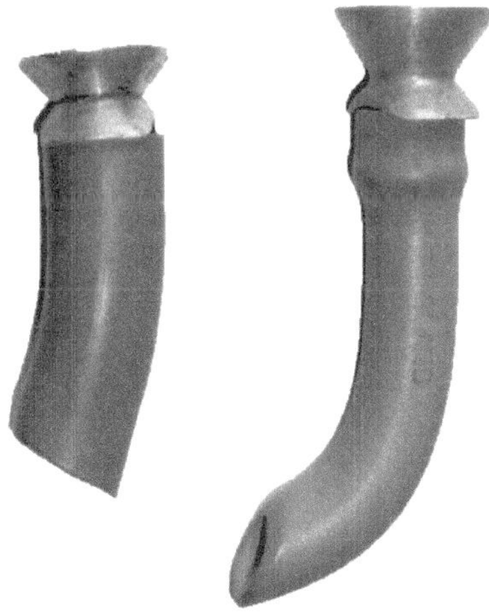

- Water's airway: Made of metal and has two holes in the sides near the pharyngeal end and right or left nipple for attachment of oxygen catheter

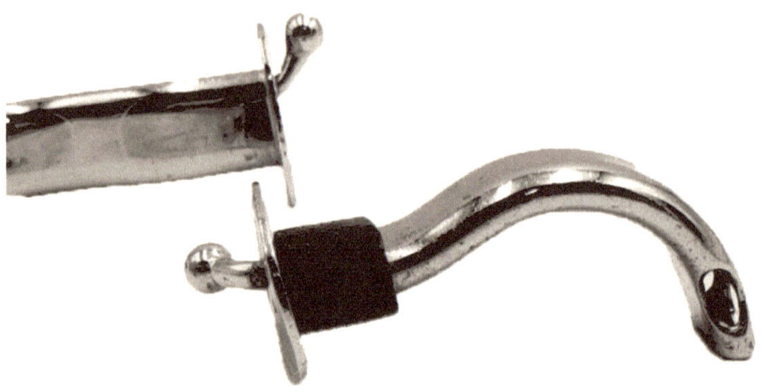

Figure 30: Water's Airway

- Guedel airway: Made of rubber, standard pharyngeal airway

Figure 31: Guedel Airway

- Complications:
  - Trauma
  - Risk of gag reflex stimulation and vomiting.

- *Note:*
  - Air channel should be as large as possible
  - Cleaning at regular intervals is essential
  - Proper size should be selected
  - Patient himself clears it away when he regains consciousness.

Nasopharyngeal Airway

- Here the airway tube is inserted through the nose into nasopharynx. The distal end should be kept just above the epiglottis and below the base of tongue
- Round curved tube, bevel usually left facing, and flange at the proximal end

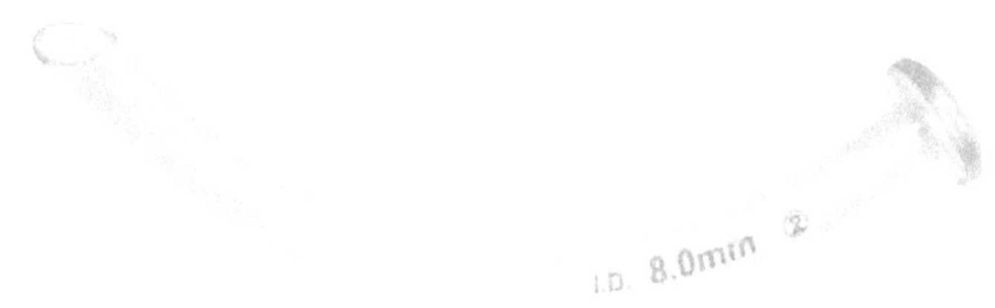

Figure 32: Nasopharyngeal Airway

- Used as an alternative to oropharyngeal airway particularly when mouth cannot be opened
- Nasotracheal suction can be done
- Better tolerated

- • Complications:
  - Injury
  - Bleeding
  - False passage.
- • Contraindications:
  - Coagulopathy
  - Nasal sepsis
  - Nasal deformity.

Laryngeal Mask Airway

- • Popularly used as alternative either to face mask or endotracheal tube for anaesthesia
- • Transparent tube with an elliptical cuff resembling small face mask. It can be inflated by a pilot balloon with a self-sealing valve. The proximal or machine end provides a standard 15mm connection. Slits at the junction between the tube and cuff prevent the epiglottis from obstructing the laryngeal mask
- • Before application, the cuff is deflated and lubricated. It is gently introduced blindly into the mouth and the cuff should lie over the laryngeal inlet. It is then inflated
- • Different sizes are available. Wide internal diameter helps reduction of flow resistance.
- • Uses:
  - As an aid in difficult intubation

-   Reinforced version can be used for head/neck surgery.

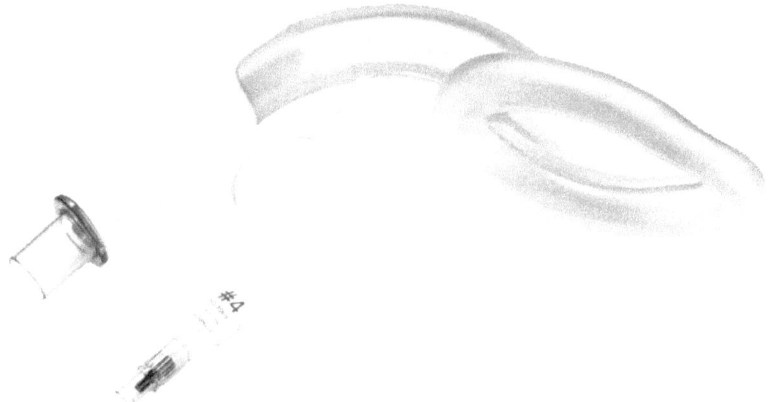

Figure 33: Laryngeal Mask Airway

Advantages:
-   Easy to apply
-   No laryngoscopy needed.

Disadvantages:
-   Does not protect against aspiration of gastric contents
-   Airway obstruction can occur
-   Less reliable and predictable than using cuffed endotracheal intubation
-   Not a substitute for tracheal intubation.
-   Contraindications:
    -   Vomiting prone patients
    -   Oropharyngeal mass/abscess.

Laryngoscopes

- Device used to perform direct laryngoscopy and to aid endotracheal intubation
- Consists of a handle and a blade. Handle provides power source/batteries. Blade is either straight or curved and is fitted in the handle. A bulb is screwed on the blade. Electrical connection occurs when the blade is opened for use

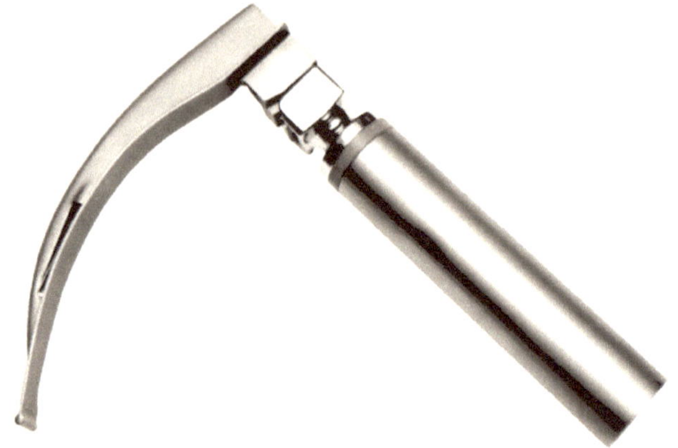

Figure 34: Laryngoscope

Various designs and shapes are available

- Straight bladed Magill laryngoscope
    - It picks up the epiglottis. Tip of the laryngoscope is advanced over the posterior border of the epiglottis and is then lifted directly to see the laryngeal inlet
    - Usually needed for intubating the neonates, infants and children. Larger blades can be used for adults.

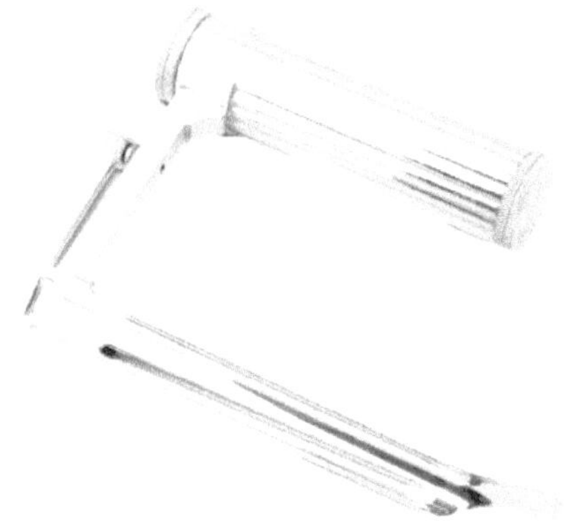

Figure 35: Straight Bladed Magill Laryngoscope

- Curved blade Macintosh laryngoscope
  - Designed to fit in the oral/oropharyngeal cavity. Usually introduced through the right angle of the oral cavity and advanced to reach the vallecula. It is then lifted upward to elevate the larynx and see the vocal cords
  - Left sided Macintosh blade is also available. It is meant for left handed anaesthetists and also in patients with right sided deformity, where the use of right sided blade insertion is difficult.
- McCoy laryngoscope
  Modified Macintosh laryngoscope with a hinged tip which is operated by lever mecha present in handle. Helpful in difficult intubation.

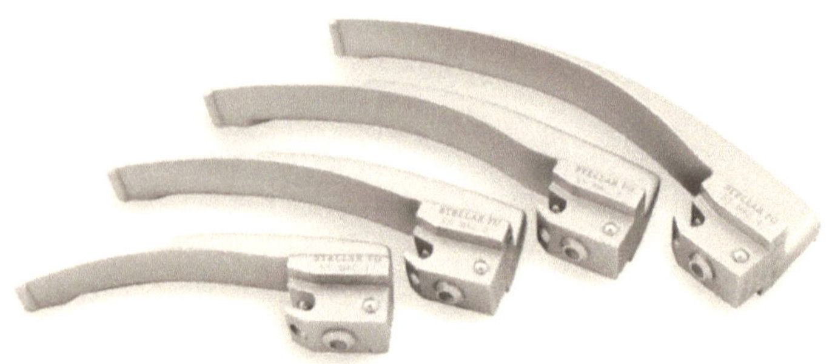

Figure 36: Macintosh Laryngoscope Blades

- Complications:
  - Trauma
  - Cardiovascular reflex disturbances
  - Malfunction.

NB: Two functional laryngoscopes should always be available 'during endotracheal intubation.

Endotracheal Tube Connections

- 15mm disposable connections provided with plastic disposable endotracheal tubes
- Variety of endotracheal connections available
  - Magill connection: Curved, one end is serrated and the other end tapered to fit catheter mount. Nasal type has a sharper curve than the oral connections. Causes less resistance to gas flows. (Figs 9.35 and 9.36)

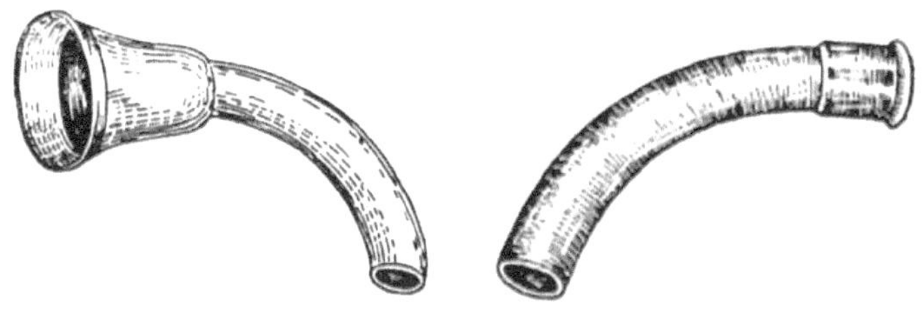

Figure 37: Magill Connection Nasal and Oral

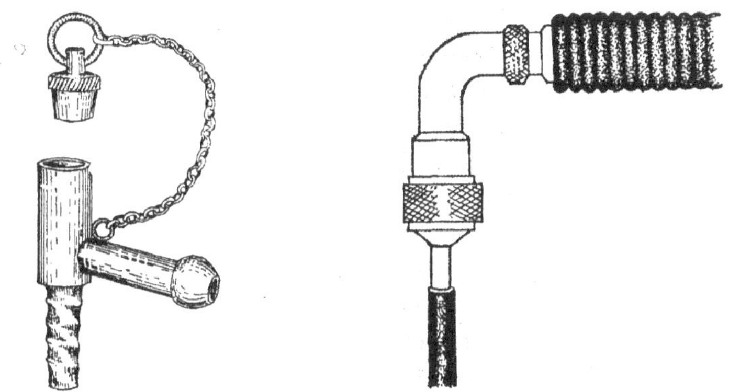

Figure 38: Cobb's Suction Union and Nosworthy Endotracheal Connection

- Rowbotham: Right angled. The end where the tracheal tube is attached is serrated and tapered
- Cobb's: Cobb's suction union is a modification of a Rowbotham connector. Designed to allow a suction catheter down the tube (Fig. 9.37)
- Nosworthy
- Worcester.

Catheter Mount

- Made of metal tube and one end provides a small rubber tube

- Machine end is metallic to be attached to the expiratory valve. Patient end attached to endotracheal tube
- Standard size
- Internal diameter wide, gas flow resistance is low
- Acts as an adaptor between endotracheal tube and breathing system
- Acts to stabilize the endotracheal tube
- Length contributes to dead space
- In some designs there is a built-in condenser humidifier.

Figure 39: Catheter Mount

Intubating Forceps (Magill)

- Used to manipulate a Nasotracheal or nasogastric tube through the oropharynx and into the correct position
- Designed to be held at right hand
- Dinner fork curvature, tip is blunt, No 'catch'
- Other uses: To introduce throat pack, to remove foreign bodies, etc.
- Caution: Not to injure tube cuff and soft tissues.

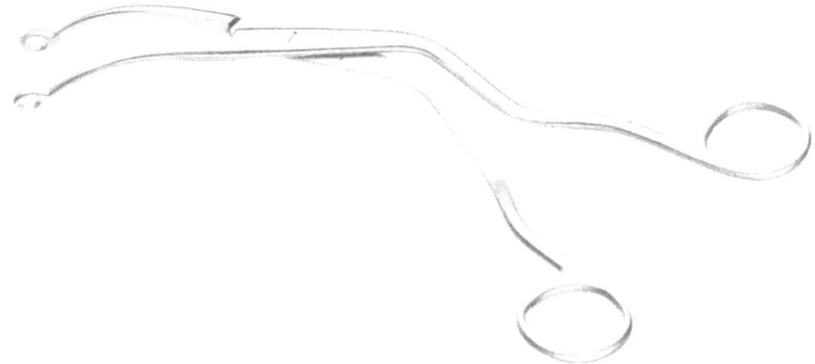

Figure 40: Magill Forceps

Laryngeal Spray

- Used to deposit a fine mist of local anaesthetic (lignocaine 4%) on the mucosa of the larynx and upper trachea
- Aids to minimize the autonomic reflexes and circulatory changes related with laryngoscopy and endotracheal intubation.

Gum Elastic Bougie

- It is used when the larynx cannot be visualized
- The bougie is inserted in the trachea through the vocal cords, then the endotracheal tube is rail roaded over it
- Bougie and the endotracheal tube should be lubricated during use.

Stylet

- The curvature of the endotracheal tube can be altered with a malleable wire or Stylet.
- It should be lubricated before use.

Ventilators

Ideal characteristics:

- Simple, portable, robust, economical
- Versatility: Tidal volume up to 1500 ml with respiration rate 60/min, variable Inspiration/Expiration (I/E) ratio. Can be used in different anaesthetic systems. Can deliver any gas/vapour
- Monitors airway pressure, inspired and exhaled minute and tidal volume, respiratory rate, inspired O_2 concentration
- Provision of humidification
- Alarms: Disconnection, high/low airway pressure, power failure
- Provision of other modes of ventilation: Positive end-expiratory pressure (PEEP), Continuous positive airway pressure (CPAP), Intermittent Mandatory Ventilation (IMV), etc.
- Easy to clean and sterilize
- Easy to use and safe
- Facilities of manual operation and emergency back-up.

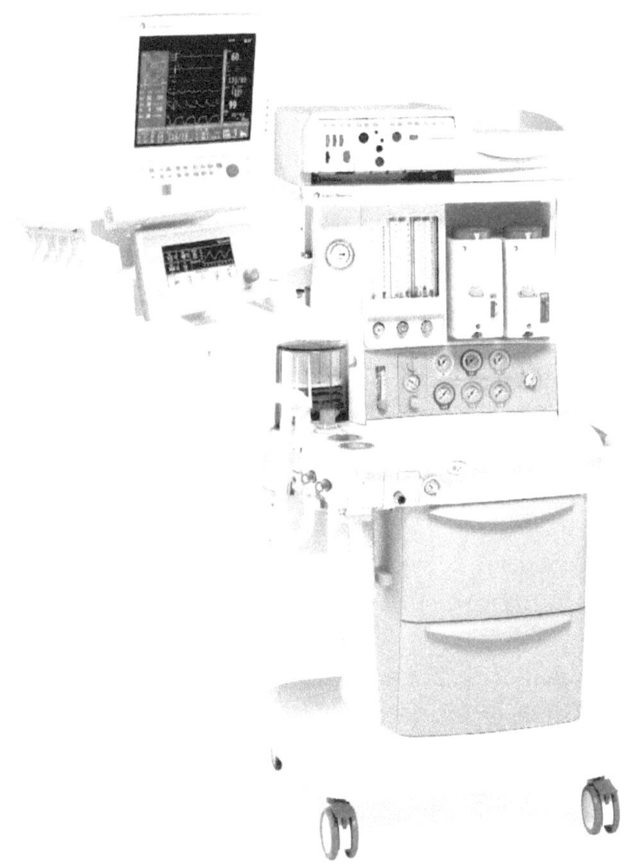

Figure 41: Anaesthesia Gas Machine Ventilator

Options:

i. Whether to use sophisticated machine with ancillary apparatus built-in or relatively simple machine with separate apparatus

ii. Ventilators suitable for Intensive Care Unit (ICU) are almost universally constant flow generators and they need to be more versatile than those in Operating Theatre (OT)

iii. Most important single feature of a satisfactory ventilator for ICU is that it can cope with changing, sometimes rapidly changing pulmonary mechanics.

Summary

Continuous-flow anaesthetic machine used to provide a measured and continuous supply of gases (oxygen, nitrous oxide, etc.), mixed with a required concentration of anesthetic vapor to the patient at a required pressure and rate. Anesthetic vaporizers vaporizes the anaesthetic Oxygen mask to deliver oxygen and/or to administer aerosolized medications
Nasal oxygen set to deliver oxygen Guedel airways hard part of the airway maintenance that connects the mouth part to the pharyngeal part
Yankauer suction tip Suction catheters used to remove secretions from the mouth, oropharynx, trachea and bronchi Peripheral venous catheter Water and sand weight bag Artificial resuscitator (Bag valve mask) manual ventilation Bain circuit respiratory maintenance circuit
Laryngoscope used to view larynx including the vocal cords, the glottis, etc.

Endotracheal tube a tube introduced into the patient's trachea to maintain a patient to ensure that air reaches the lungs for respiration Laryngeal mask airway (LMA) a less stimulating alternative to an endotracheal tube Endoscope to look inside the larynx, trachea, bronchi
Eschmann stylet or Gum elastic bougie a flexible device introduced through the mouth during some intubation procedures;

if the stylet is in the trachea, while passing in, gives a sensation of bumps and then finally stops going in at a point, it indicates that it was gliding over tracheal rings and has stopped at one of the bronchi (the patient may even cough during this time); if it goes into the esophagus, it will not bump and neither will it stop going in; used to judge where the endotracheal tube has gone in

HEPA Filter- to filter out dust particles from the gas being given to the patient Hypodermic needle for injections, infusions, etc. Tuohy needle for epidural catheter insertion Spinal needle used for puncturing the spinal canal for injection of medications in spinal anaesthesia Epidural catheter used to administer medications into the epidural space Syringe to inject medications Mucus sucker to aspirate any fluid specially mucus from the respiratory passage Variable performance devices

Fixed performance devices Peripheral Nerve Stimulator to locate the nerve during Regional Anesthesia TOF Monitor to decide the repeat / reverse the Anesthesia effect General anaesthesia does not always require the anaesthetic machine, tested daily, as basic equipment. Anesthesia machines may differ in appearance, size and degree of sophistication but generally speaking, they consist of sections for: Ventilation Peripheral Nerve Stimulator space for monitoring equipment accessories storage space worktop

It is imperative that essential medical pipeline gas supply, e.g. oxygen, nitrous oxide and air, are secured firmly to the machine, and readily available without any obstructions, defects or pressure leaks. They should also be checked in between cases, ensuring that the breathing apparatus and breathing circuit are fully patent, for the safe anaesthesia of patients. Major manufacturers of anaesthetic machines are General Electric (GE), Larsen & Toubro Limited, Draeger and MAQUET.

Bibliography

Aridi M, Hussein B, Hajj-Hassan M, Khachfe HM. . (2016). *A novel approach for healthcare equipment lifespan assessment. .* Int J Adv Life Sci. 2016;8:1-15.

Bodman R, Gillies D. Harold Griffith. . (1992). *The evolution of modern anaesthesia. .* Toronto: Hannah Institute, : Oxford: Dundurn Press; 1992.

Brockwell RC, Andrews GG. . (2002). *Understanding Your Anaesthesia Machine;.* Philadelphia: ASA Refresher Courses. Vol. 4. Pennsylvania: Lippincott Williams and Wilkins;pp. 41–59. .

Kalu Q, Edentekhe TA, Eguma S. (2020). *Anesthesia equipment and their chain of survival.* Calabar J Health Sci 2020;4(1):13-9.

Mutia D, Kihiu J, Maranga S. . (2012). *Maintenance management of medical equipment in hospitals. .* Ind Eng Lett. 2012;2:5-19.

Neumar RW, Shuster M, Callaway CW, Gent LM, Atkins DL, Bhanji F. . (2015). *American heart association guidelines update for cardiopulmonary resuscitation and emergency cardiovascular care. .* Part 1: Executive summary: Circulation. 2015;132:S315-67.

SECTION TWO:
ANAESTHETIC MACHINE

The anesthetic machine is a sophisticated assembly of equipment rather than a device that produces anesthetics. A gas mixing and delivery system, an anesthetic breathing system (circuit), a ventilator, and a variety of monitors make up its three main parts. Some recently created devices, known as anesthesia workstations, feature extremely intricate integrated electrical systems.

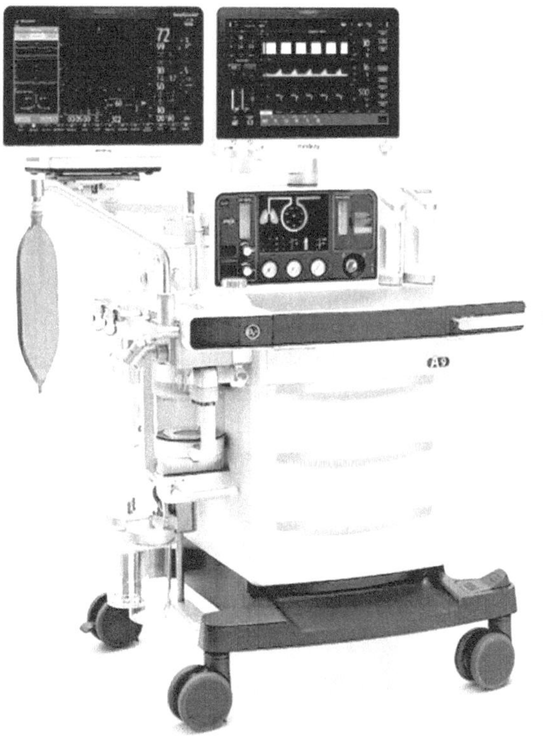

A supply of purified gases is linked to the anesthetic machine. Numerous devices also have a source of compressed air, and these gases frequently comprise oxygen and nitrous oxide. The precise concentrations are ensured and the minimal amount of oxygen that can be utilized are limited thanks to the specific mechanism that mixes all the gases. The anesthetist can add one of a variety of additional, more potent anesthetic agents—known as inhalational agents—to this gas mixture. These start off as liquids and are put in a vaporizer, which turns them into gases and adds them to the gas mixture in precisely measured concentrations.

Components of Anaesthetic Machine:

- O2 and anaesthetic gas supply
- Pressure gauges
- Reducing valve
- Flow meters
- Vapourizers
- Common gas outlet
- Other features such as O_2 flush, pressure relief valve, O_2 supply failure alarm, suction apparatus.
- Monitoring devices, mechanical ventilator, breathing system.

Safety Devices incorporated in the anaesthetic machine
- Gas supplies pipeline, cylinders
- Flow meters e.g. flullor, off position, control knob,
- Vapourizers
- Fresh gas delivery: Breathing system and ventilators
- Scavenging
- Monitoring
- Pressure regulators
- Pressure relief device

- Diameter index safety (Non-interchangeable screw thread) system (pin index).
- Hose pipes to make them kink proof.
- Oxygen failure warning devices
- Oxygen flush
- Tubes has antistatic coating to prevent bobbing from sticking.
- Visible bobbing throughout the length of tube
- Mandatory minimum O_2 flow e.g. 50 – 250ml to prevent hypoxia.
- Oxygen alarm
- Keyed and colour coded vapourizer filling system
- Vaporizers interlock
- Main on/off switch for electrical power to integral monitors and alarms.
- Air pressure alarm.

Explain uses of O_2 in the Anaesthetic machine
- Camer gas for inhalational anaesthetic agents
- Pre-oxygenation before induction of anaesthetic
- To maintain saturation of blood during surgery.
- Used for IPPV
- Entonox for obstetric analgesia in labour.
- Prevent hypoxia (Treat hypoxia)
- Prevent surgical site infection
- To ease pain after surgery
- Facilitates physical therapy.

Temperature Compensated Vaporizer
e.g. (i) Epstein Macintosh Oxford (EMO)

- Variables by pass
- Incomplete vaporization – Draw over V_x

- Flow over without wicks
- Low resistance
- Agent – specific for Ether
- Temperature compensated by bellows
- Temperature stabilized by water jacket
- Transportable but heavy (10Kg)

OR

e.g (ii) Fluotec Mkz (Fmz),

- Variable by pass
- Flow over with wicks
- Low resistance; agent specific Halothane
- Temperature compensated with bimetallic strip
- Non-tippable
- No interlocks
- Non-keyed filler
- Subject to pumping and pressuring effect.

Temperature uncompensated vapourizer (Not temperature compensated)

i) Oxford Miniative Vapourizer (OMV)

- Variable bypass
- Flow over with metal mesh wicks
- Low resistance
- Multiple agents
- Not temperature compsenated
- Light weight
- Chamber contains only 50ml of agent
- Cooling limits maximum output to 2-4% with halothane
- Two units in series required for a seroflourane induction
- Can be used with self-infalting bag or with an EMO.

Modern – Plenum Vapourizer Temperature compensated.

- Driven by positive pressure from the anaesthetic massive
- Performance is instant for spontaneous or mechanical breathing ventilation.
- Internal resistance is high but can be caliberated to deliver accurately a precise concentration of volatile vapour
- A reliable elegant device.
- Works for many hundreds of homes
- Requires very little maintenance
- Output 1-2%.
- Works within a specific temperature range (compensatory)
- Metallic jacket 5kg weight.
- Entrance control by a bimetallic strip.

Signs of Electrolyte Imbalance

- Nausea
- Vomiting
- Diarrhea or conspitation
- Irregular heartbeat
- Tarchycandia
- Fatigue
- Lethargy
- Convulsions or seizures
- Abdominal cramping
- Muscle cramping
- Irritability
- Headaches
- Confusion
- Numbness and fingling

Peri Operative Embolism

- Acute pulmonary embolism and venous thromboses e.g the peri operative embolism
- Potentially fatal complication during perioperative period.
- Early diagnosis and treatment prevent imorbidity and mortality.
- Preventing measure anticoagulant
- Fast detection, correct diagnosis and appropriate treatment overcome this severe complication.
- Employ techniques that target embolism directly is essential.

Management: - Vasopressors, inotopes

- Mechanical ventilator can stabilize patients
- Thrombolytic therapy improves pulmonary perfusion
- And reduce pulmonary artery pressure
- Surgical embolectomy and catheter-based therapies is yet to be fully defined.

Isoflurane

Approved for medical use in 1979.

- Trade name is Forane – Halogenated other family medication
- Inhalational anaesthetic agent
- For maintenance of general anaesthetic
- Irritate airway
- Is very effective – comes in bottle of 250ml

Side effect – Respiratory depression, low blood pressure
- Irregular heart beat
- Malignant hyperthermia
- Hyper kalaemia

Uses:

- Is adrainster with air or pure oxygen
- Physical properties induce anaesthesia more rapid than halothane.

Adverse Effect

- Risk of neuro degeneration increase
- Risk for brain damage – Alzbomers disease

Physical Properties: Molecular weight 184.5glmol

- Boiling point (at 1 atm): 48.5°C
- Density (at at 25^0C): 1.496 glml
- MAC – 1.15vol%
- Vapour – 238 mmHg 31.7kpa (at 20^0C), 450mmHG 60.0kpa (at 35^0C)
- Water solubility 13.5mm (at 25^0C)
- Blood gas partition coefficient: 1.4
- Oil gas partition coefficient – 98
- A racemic mixture of (R) and (S) optical isomers
- Vaporizes readily, liquid at room temperature
- It does not burn.

Mechanism of Action:

- Reduces pain sensitivity (analgesia)
- Relaxes muscles
- Build to GABA, glutamate and glycine receptors
- Act as a positive allosteric modulator of GABA
- Potentiate glyane receptor which decreases moto function
- Inhibit conduction in activated potassium channels.
- Affects intracellular molecules
- Activates calcium ATpase by increasing membrane fluidity.
- Bind to D submit of ATP synthesis and NADA dehydrogenase

- Reduces plasma endocannabinoid AEA concentrations after loss of consciousness.

Premedication

- Administration of medication before Anaesthetic
- To prepare patient for anaesthetics
- To provide optimal conditions for surgery this include
- Reducing anxiety, Amnesia and pain
- Promote amnesia
- Reduce secretions
- Reduce volume of PH of gastric contents (to avoid mendelson syndrome)
- Reduce post operative nausea and vomiting
- Enhance hypnotic effects of G.A.
- Reduce vagal reflexes to intubation

Specific Indications:

Prevention of ineffective endocarditis.

- Is given 1.m or 1.v and orally for children and those with bleeding disorders
- Premedication is given 1 – 3 loms preoperatively.
- Topical anaesthetic e.g EMLA are often prescribed for children before cannulation.
- Pre medication - anticholinagics, analgesic hyosanie are used

Factors that Reduces Sedative Premedication

- Increasing use of day-case surgery
- Same day admission where pt do not find abed until just after surgery.
- Changes to the surgical list, make the timing of drug delivery difficult.

- Choice of drugs used for premedication depends on the procedure, patients and anaesthetic technique.

Example of premedications

- Benzodiazepines (Diazipam, midazolam, temazepam lorazepam)
- Analgesic: Opoids, Murpine, pethidine, fentanyl citrate, pentazosine, pcm, Nos AIO.
- Oral anti unistamines for children e.g Promethazine
- Antivogal (Anti – Sialogogues e.g Glycopyrotate)
- Anti emetics – butyro phenones, hyoscine, metoclopramide
- H_2 – receptor antagonist or proton e.g. Rinitchin, Omeprazole. 15 – 30 Minutes 64 induction.

Summary

Medical gases (oxygen, nitrous oxide, and air) are delivered under pressure to the anesthetic machine, which precisely regulates the flow of each gas separately. Prior to adding a known concentration of an inhalational agent vapour, a gas mixture with the required composition and flow rate is first generated. Fresh gas flow (FGF), as well as gas and vapour mixes for the patient's breathing system, are continually fed to the machine's common gas output.

Gas supplies, pressure gauges, pressure regulators (reduction valves), flow meters, vaporizers, common gas outlets, and a number of additional features, such as high-flow oxygen flush, pressure relief valve, oxygen supply failure warning, and suction apparatus, are all included in it. The majority of current anesthesia devices or stations include a bag-in-bottle ventilator and a circular breathing system.

References

Bodman R, Gillies D. Harold Griffith. . (1992). *The evolution of modern anaesthesia. .* Toronto: Hannah Institute, : Oxford: Dundurn Press; 1992.

Brockwell RC, Andrews GG. . (2002). *Understanding Your Anaesthesia Machine;.* Philadelphia: ASA Refresher Courses. Vol. 4. Pennsylvania: Lippincott Williams and Wilkins;pp. 41–59. .

Kalu Q, Edentekhe TA, Eguma S. (2020). *Anesthesia equipment and their chain of survival.* Calabar J Health Sci 2020;4(1):13-9.

MS., P. (1985). *A calculus of suffering: pain, professionalism and anesthesia in nineteenth-century America.* New York, NY: Columbia University Press; 1985; p. 421. .

Mutia D, Kihiu J, Maranga S. . (2012). *Maintenance management of medical equipment in hospitals. .* Ind Eng Lett. 2012;2:5-19.

9 783384 379146